Vitality of Life

Anna Baker

Anna Baker

Copyright holder: © 2024 Andrea Jimenez
Author: © Anna Baker

Legal and Copyright Information

This book may not be reproduced, distributed, or transmitted in any form or by any means, electronic or mechanical, including photocopying, recording, or any information storage and retrieval system, without the prior written permission of the author.

First edition
All Rights Reserved

Index

Anna Baker

The Art of Living in the Present

Living in the present is one of the most fundamental principles to achieve a full and satisfying life. However, in a world where distractions are constant and the pace of life is increasingly accelerated, it can be difficult to keep our attention in the here and now. The mind has a natural tendency to wander, whether remembering the past or anticipating the future, which often prevents us from fully enjoying the present moment. Learning to live in the present does not mean ignoring our responsibilities or stopping planning for the future, but rather it is about being fully aware and committed to what we are doing at every moment.

The practice of living in the present, also known as mindfulness, is a skill that can be developed over time. Often, we don't realize how distracted we are until we try to focus on the current moment. A simple exercise to begin developing this skill is to pay attention to your breathing. Breathing is one of the most basic and essential functions of life, and yet, most of the time we do it automatically, without thinking about it. By focusing on our breathing, consciously inhaling and exhaling, we can begin to anchor our mind in the present.

Another important aspect of living in the present is acceptance. Accepting the moment as it is, without judging it or trying to change it, allows us to experience life in a more fulfilling and less stressful way. This does not mean that we should resign ourselves to negative circumstances, but rather that we should recognize them without resistance and decide how to consciously respond. We often fight against reality when it is not as we wish, which only increases our suffering. By accepting what is, we can find peace and clarity to make more effective decisions.

Mindfulness also extends to our interactions with others. Too often, while we are in a conversation, our minds race ahead, thinking about what we are going to say next or getting distracted by other thoughts. This can cause us to miss important details of the conversation and not be truly present for the other person. Practicing active listening, paying all our attention to the person who is speaking and without internal interruptions, improves the quality of our relationships and allows us to connect more deeply with others.

The environment also plays a crucial role in our ability to live in the present. Many times, our spaces are full of clutter and objects that distract us. Creating an orderly and calm environment can facilitate focus and peace of mind. Plus, spending time in nature is a powerful way to reconnect with the present. Nature, with its slow and steady rhythm, reminds us of the importance of simplicity and invites us to be more aware of our senses and the wonders that surround us.

A significant benefit of living in the present is stress reduction. Most of our stress comes from worrying about the future or regretting the past. By focusing our attention on what is happening right now, we can reduce those worries and feel calmer. This does not mean that we ignore problems or challenges, but rather that we approach them with a clear and focused mind, which often leads to more effective solutions.

Living in the present also improves our ability to enjoy life. Moments of happiness and joy are often fleeting, and if we are distracted or worried, we can miss the opportunity to fully enjoy them. By being present, we can savor every moment, from the simplest to the most extraordinary, and create richer, more meaningful memories.

Finally, living in the present allows us to be more aware of ourselves. By paying attention to our thoughts, emotions, and actions as they occur, we develop greater self-awareness. This self-awareness is essential for personal growth, as it allows us to identify patterns of behavior and thinking that may be unhealthy and make the necessary changes to improve our lives.

In short, the art of living in the present is a skill that requires practice and patience, but offers significant rewards in terms of well-being and personal satisfaction. By learning to focus on the here and now, to accept reality without resistance, and to participate fully in our experiences, we can lead richer, more meaningful lives. Living in the present is, ultimately, the key to enjoying each day to the fullest and to finding peace and happiness in everyday life.

Happiness in Everyday Life

Happiness is a concept that often seems elusive, as if it were reserved for special moments or extraordinary achievements. However, true happiness is not found in great events or ideal circumstances; It is found in the small details and simple joys we experience every day. Learning to recognize and appreciate these little things is key to living a fuller and more satisfying life. Happiness in everyday life is something that we can all cultivate, regardless of our circumstances, and doing so can transform our perception of life.

One of the first steps to finding happiness in everyday life is to change our perspective. We are often so focused on what we don't have or what we are missing that we forget what is already present in our lives. This focus on lack leads us to ignore the little things that could bring joy and satisfaction. For example, the simple fact of enjoying a cup of coffee in the morning, listening to the birds sing, or feeling the warmth of the sun on our skin are moments of happiness that, if we consciously appreciate them, can improve our state. mood and general well-being.

Gratitude is a powerful tool to find happiness in everyday life. When we practice gratitude, we train our minds to focus on the positive. This does not mean that we should ignore challenges or difficulties, but rather that we should actively look for the things we can be grateful for, no matter how small. Keeping a gratitude journal, in which we write down three things we appreciate each day, is a simple but effective practice that can help us reorient our minds toward the positive side of life. This daily practice not only increases our happiness, but also makes us more resilient in the face of adversity.

Another way to find happiness in everyday life is through connection with others. Human relationships are a deep source of joy, and it is often the small gestures of kindness and caring that count most. A hug, a smile, a sincere conversation with a friend or loved one, are moments that can fill our days with warmth and satisfaction. Taking time to strengthen our relationships, actively listen, and be present for others not only enriches our lives, but also connects us to a sense of community and belonging.

The act of taking care of ourselves is also a source of everyday happiness. This can include simple practices like taking a relaxing bath, reading a book we like, or taking a walk in the park. These small actions, when done with intention and without haste, allow us to reconnect with ourselves and recharge our energies. Many times, in our daily routine, we forget the importance of giving ourselves small moments of self-care, but by doing so, we are cultivating a space for happiness in our lives.

Furthermore, the art of enjoying what we do, even in the most mundane tasks, is another path to everyday happiness. We often get caught up in the idea that certain activities are tedious or boring. However, if we approach these tasks with a positive attitude and full attention, we can find satisfaction even in them. For example, cooking a meal for ourselves or our family can become a moment of creativity and connection if we take the time to enjoy the process. In the same way, tidying up the house can be an act of caring, not only for the space, but also for ourselves, by creating a more harmonious and pleasant environment.

The ability to find happiness in the everyday is also closely related to simplicity. We live in a world where we are often encouraged to seek more: more things, more experiences, more achievements. However, the constant search for more can cause us to overlook the joy found in the simple. Learning to simplify our lives, reduce clutter, both physical and mental, and focus on what really matters allows us to experience happiness in a more consistent and accessible way. Sometimes, it is in the simplest moments, like sitting quietly watching a sunset, where we find the greatest peace and happiness.

Finally, it is important to remember that happiness in everyday life is not a state of constant joy or perfection. Rather, it is a willingness to appreciate the good in our lives, even when not everything is ideal. It is a daily practice of mindfulness and gratitude, a commitment to see the beauty in the ordinary and to value the small moments that, when added up, make up the majority of our lives. Happiness, then, is not something we have to wait for, but something we can find every day, in the smallest details and in the simplest experiences.

In short, happiness in everyday life is a choice, an attitude that we can develop by paying attention to the little things around us and by cultivating gratitude and connection with ourselves and others. By doing so, we discover that life is full of moments of joy, and that true happiness is not in what we hope for or what we desire, but in what we already have, in what we live day by day.

Nutrition for Body and Soul

Nutrition is fundamental to our well-being, and it refers not only to the food we consume, but also how we nourish our mind and spirit. The way we care for our body and mind directly influences our physical and emotional health, so it's important to pay attention to the simplest aspects of nutrition, both for body and soul. This chapter addresses how we can improve our quality of life through a balanced diet and practices that nourish our spirit, offering a holistic vision of well-being.

Starting with the body, food is the basis of a healthy life. What we eat affects our energy, our concentration and, in general, our mood. A balanced diet is key to maintaining a strong body and a clear mind. This doesn't mean we should follow a strict diet or deprive ourselves of foods we enjoy, but it's about finding a balance that works for us. Including a variety of fresh, natural foods in our diet, such as fruits, vegetables, whole grains and quality proteins, provides us with the nutrients we need to function optimally. These foods are rich in vitamins, minerals and antioxidants that not only keep us healthy, but can also improve our skin, strengthen our immune system and increase our vitality.

It is also important to remember that each body is unique and what works for one person may not be right for another. Listening to our body is essential to understand which foods make us feel good and which don't. Sometimes this may involve making adjustments to our diet, such as reducing our consumption of refined sugars or processed foods, which may be tempting but, in the long term, do not provide much nutritional value. On the other hand, it is vital not to fall into the trap of extreme diets or food fads that promise quick results but can be unsustainable and unhealthy. Instead, the key is to adopt eating habits that we can maintain over time, and that help us feel good both inside and out.

But nutrition is not just about what we eat, it is also about how we eat. Eating mindfully, that is, paying attention to what we are eating and enjoying each bite, can improve our relationship with food and our digestion. Instead of eating in a hurry or distractedly, sitting at the table and savoring food without rushing helps us connect with our body and be more aware of the signals of hunger and satiety. This not only improves our digestion, but also allows us to enjoy food more and feel more satisfied with what we eat. Plus, when we eat mindfully, we're more likely to make food choices that truly nourish our bodies and make us feel good.

Just as it is important to nourish our body, it is also important to nourish our soul. This means taking care of our emotional and mental well-being, which is as vital as maintaining a balanced diet. How we nourish our soul can vary from person to person, but it generally involves doing things that fill us with joy, peace, and satisfaction. This can include activities like reading a good book, spending time in nature, practicing meditation, or simply enjoying the company of loved ones. These activities allow us to disconnect from daily stress and reconnect with what really matters in life, providing us with a deep and lasting sense of well-being.

Self-care is another essential way to nourish our soul. This can be as simple as taking a few minutes a day to relax, breathe deeply, or reflect on what we are grateful for. Taking care of ourselves is not a selfish act, but a necessity to maintain our emotional balance and mental health. When we take the time to nourish our soul, we become more resilient to life's challenges and more able to enjoy happy moments. Additionally, when we are good for ourselves, we can also be better for others, offering our love and support in a more authentic and generous way.

Finally, nourishment of the body and soul are deeply interconnected. When we take care of our body through good nutrition, we feel better physically and emotionally, which in turn allows us to nourish our soul more easily. Likewise, when our spirit is well nourished, it is easier to make healthy choices for our body as we are more in tune with our needs and desires. This positive cycle of mutual care between body and soul is what allows us to live a full and satisfying life.

In conclusion, nourishing the body and soul is a daily practice that requires attention and care. It is not about seeking perfection, but about finding a balance that allows us to feel good in all aspects of our life. By adopting a balanced and conscious diet, and taking the time necessary to care for our emotional well-being, we can significantly improve our quality of life. This holistic nutrition not only helps us stay healthy, but also allows us to enjoy life more, appreciate the simple moments, and find lasting happiness in our daily lives.

Exercise and Wellness

Exercise is one of the fundamental pillars to maintain a healthy and balanced lifestyle. However, it is often associated with something that must be done out of obligation or to achieve certain physical goals, such as losing weight or gaining muscle mass. While these may be added benefits, exercise is much more than that. It is a powerful tool to improve not only our physical health, but also our mental and emotional well-being. Understanding exercise as a form of self-care, rather than a task or a means to an end, can transform our relationship with it and motivate us to integrate it more naturally into our daily lives.

Exercise, in its simplest form, is movement. Our body is designed to move, and when we do, we unleash a series of benefits that go beyond what we can see with the naked eye. When we move, whether walking, dancing, running or practicing yoga, we are strengthening our heart, improving our circulation, and helping to keep our muscles and joints in good condition. But movement also has a profound impact on our minds. Numerous studies have shown that regular exercise can reduce levels of stress, anxiety and depression. This is because when we exercise, our brain releases endorphins, often known as the "happy hormones", which improve our mood and make us feel more positive and energized.

Exercise doesn't have to be complicated or time-consuming to be effective. Sometimes the thought of spending hours in a gym may seem daunting, but it's not necessary. Incorporating small moments of physical activity throughout the day can have a significant impact on our overall well-being. For example, walking for 30 minutes a day, whether in a park, in the city or even inside the house, can be enough to improve our cardiovascular and mental health. The important thing is to find an activity that we enjoy and that we can do consistently. The key is to move regularly, not to exercise intensely only occasionally.

In addition to the physical and mental benefits, exercise can also be a way to connect with ourselves and our environment. Activities like yoga or tai chi, for example, combine movement with conscious breathing and meditation, which not only strengthens the body, but also calms the mind and balances emotions. These practices invite us to be more aware of our body, to listen to its signals and respect its limits, which is essential to maintain a healthy balance. Even more dynamic activities, such as running or swimming, can become moments of active reflection and meditation, if we allow ourselves to enjoy the process instead of focusing solely on the result.

Exercise can also be an excellent opportunity to socialize and strengthen our relationships. Participating in group physical activities, such as dance classes, community walks, or team sports, allows us to share quality time with others, which enriches our lives and gives us a sense of community. These social interactions not only make exercise more fun and motivating, but they also provide us with emotional support, which is crucial for our well-being. By surrounding ourselves with people with similar interests, we create a positive environment that encourages us to remain active and committed to our health.

Another important aspect to consider is that exercise should not be seen as a form of punishment or as something we do solely to "compensate" for what we eat. This mindset can create an unhealthy relationship with physical activity and our bodies. Instead, we should see exercise as an act of love toward ourselves, a way to care for our body and mind. By shifting our perspective and focusing on how we feel after exercising, rather than how we look, we can begin to enjoy the process more and incorporate movement into our daily lives in a more natural and sustainable way.

For many people, one of the biggest challenges is finding the time to exercise. In a busy daily routine, it may seem difficult to dedicate an hour a day to physical activity. However, exercise doesn't have to be a separate activity from the rest of our day. We can incorporate movement into our daily activities in creative ways. For example, choosing to take the stairs instead of the elevator, walking or cycling instead of driving, or even stretching while watching TV, are small actions that can add up to big benefits over time. The idea is to look for opportunities to move throughout the day, rather than viewing exercise as something we can only do in a gym or class.

Finally, it is important to remember that exercise should be a pleasurable experience. We don't all enjoy the same activities, and it's okay to experiment with different types of exercise until you find what you really like. For some, it may be hiking in nature; For others, it may be dance, yoga, or even gardening. What matters is that we move in a way that makes us feel good, that allows us to enjoy the moment and that contributes to our overall well-being. By adopting this attitude towards exercise, we will see it not as an obligation, but as an integral part of our life that enriches our body, our mind and our spirit.

In short, exercise and wellness are intrinsically connected. Through movement, we not only improve our physical health, but we also cultivate a more positive state of mind and emotional balance. By finding ways to integrate exercise into our daily lives, in ways that are enjoyable and sustainable, we can transform our relationship with movement and, consequently, our well-being. Exercise is a powerful form of self-care, and when we approach it with an attitude of love and gratitude toward our bodies, it allows us to live more fully and healthily every day.

The Importance of Sleep

Sleep is a fundamental pillar for our health and well-being, although we often underestimate it in our daily lives. In a world that values productivity and constant activity, sleep can seem like a waste of time, something that is sacrificed in order to get more done. However, the reality is that sleep is essential for our body and mind. Sleep is not just a moment of passive rest; It is an active process during which the body and brain perform crucial functions that could not be carried out while we are awake. Understanding the importance of sleep and how it affects all aspects of our lives is key to living in a healthy and balanced way.

First of all, sleep is the time when our body regenerates. During sleeping hours, the body works to repair tissues, build bones and muscles, and strengthen the immune system. These functions are vital to keeping us healthy and resistant to illness and injury. Without adequate sleep, these processes are disrupted, which can lead to increased susceptibility to illness, increased stress, and slower recovery from any ailments or physical fatigue. Additionally, sleep also helps regulate many of the body's hormones, including those that control appetite and metabolism, meaning that getting enough sleep can help maintain a healthy weight and avoid long-term metabolic problems.

Sleep is also essential for mental health. During the night, the brain processes and organizes the information it has received during the day. This includes consolidating memory, solving problems, and eliminating toxins that have accumulated during waking hours. Without adequate sleep, this process is compromised, which can lead to memory problems, difficulty concentrating, and a decrease in decision-making ability. In the long term, lack of sleep has been linked to an increased risk of developing mental disorders such as depression and anxiety. Therefore, sleep is a fundamental part of our emotional and mental health, and is necessary to maintain a clear and balanced mind.

One of the most important aspects of sleep is quantity and quality. It is not only important to get a sufficient number of hours of sleep each night, but also to ensure that those hours are quality hours. This means we must go through the different phases of sleep, including deep sleep and REM (rapid eye movement) sleep, which are crucial for physical and mental restoration. Unfortunately, many of us have trouble getting adequate sleep due to factors such as stress, excessive use of electronic devices before bed, or an unfavorable sleep environment. These factors can disrupt sleep or cause it to not be deep enough, leaving us feeling tired and less able to cope with the demands of the next day.

To improve sleep quality, it is important to establish a regular sleep routine. Going to bed and waking up at the same time every day, even on weekends, helps regulate the body's biological clock, known as the circadian rhythm. This internal clock controls the sleep-wake cycle and is influenced by external factors such as light. Maintaining a regular routine helps your body know when it's time to sleep and when it's time to wake up, making it easier to fall asleep and rest more effectively. Additionally, creating an environment conducive to sleep, such as a dark, quiet, and cool room, can significantly improve sleep quality.

Another important aspect is preparation before going to sleep. Activities such as reading a book, taking a hot bath, or practicing relaxation techniques such as deep breathing or meditation can help calm the mind and prepare the body for sleep. It is essential to avoid using electronic devices at least an hour before bedtime, as the blue light emitted by screens can interfere with the production of melatonin, the hormone that regulates sleep. Instead, it is better to opt for activities that relax us and help us disconnect from the worries of the day. It is also important to avoid consuming heavy foods, caffeine or alcohol before bed, as these can interfere with the quality of sleep.

The impact of sleep on our mood and our ability to manage stress is also significant. When we don't get enough sleep, we are more likely to feel irritable, anxious, and less able to handle stressful situations. This is because sleep plays a crucial role in regulating our emotions. During sleep, the brain processes and balances emotions, allowing us to respond more calmly and rationally to the challenges we face during the day. Sleeping well, therefore, not only helps us feel better physically, but also to be more emotionally balanced and have a better ability to face difficulties.

Finally, it is important to recognize that sleep is an integral part of self-care. We often prioritize other activities over sleep, such as working longer hours, socializing, or simply spending time on leisure activities. While these activities are important, they should not come at the expense of getting a good night's rest. Getting enough sleep is one of the simplest and most effective ways to take care of ourselves. It is an act of self-love, and by doing so, we ensure that we are in the best shape possible to enjoy life and to be productive and happy.

In conclusion, sleep is essential for our physical, mental and emotional health. Sleeping well helps us maintain a strong body, a clear mind, and a balanced mood. By giving sleep the importance it deserves, and by making adjustments to our daily routine to improve both the quantity and quality of our rest, we can significantly improve our quality of life. Sleep is not a luxury, it is a necessity, and by prioritizing it, we ensure that we are taking care of ourselves in the best way possible.

Relationships and Support

Human relationships are one of the most important elements in our lives. From the moment we are born, we are surrounded by people who influence our development, well-being and happiness. These relationships are not limited to family, but include friends, colleagues, partners, and members of our community. Human connections provide us with support, a sense of belonging, and a source of joy that we could hardly find anywhere else. However, maintaining healthy relationships requires effort, communication, and mutual understanding. This chapter explores the importance of relationships and emotional support, and how these elements are fundamental to our well-being.

The human being is a social creature by nature. Since ancient times, we have depended on the community to survive. Although society has changed and evolved, the need to be connected with others remains the same. Healthy relationships give us a sense of security and help us face life's challenges with greater resilience. When we have the support of people who love and care about us, we feel better able to manage stress, overcome difficulties, and celebrate our achievements. This support can come in many forms, from a comforting conversation to practical help in times of need.

One of the most valuable aspects of relationships is emotional support. Having someone with whom to share our worries, joys and fears allows us to release tension and feel understood. Empathy, the ability to put yourself in someone else's shoes and understand their feelings, is an essential quality in any relationship. When we feel heard and understood, our emotional load is lightened, and we feel more connected to the person who provides us with that support. This type of deep connection strengthens the bonds between people and creates a solid foundation for a long-lasting relationship.

However, not all relationships are easy. Sometimes conflicts, misunderstandings, or differences arise that can test our connections with others. It is in these moments that open and honest communication becomes crucial. Expressing our feelings and needs clearly and respectfully is essential to solving problems and preventing tensions from accumulating. The skill of active listening, that is, paying genuine attention to what the other person is saying without interrupting or judging, is equally important. When both parties feel heard and valued, a mutually satisfactory solution is more likely to be reached.

In addition to emotional support, relationships also offer us a sense of belonging. Feeling like we're part of a group, whether it's a family, a circle of friends, or a community, gives us purpose and makes us feel like we're not alone. This sense of belonging is essential for our mental health, as it reduces the feeling of isolation and loneliness. Loneliness, especially when prolonged, can have negative effects on our emotional health, leading to problems such as depression and anxiety. Therefore, it is important to cultivate and maintain relationships that make us feel connected and supported.

Mutual support is also a vital aspect of relationships. Healthy relationships are based on give and take. When we help others, whether by offering advice, a helping hand, or simply being present, we not only strengthen the relationship, but we also feel good about ourselves. This exchange of support creates a positive cycle where both parties benefit and the relationship is enriched. It's important to remember that while receiving support is crucial, being able to offer it is equally valuable. Being a good friend, partner, or family member means being willing to be there for others when they need you.

Relationships also help us grow and develop as people. Through our interactions with others, we learn about ourselves, our strengths and weaknesses, and how we can improve. The challenges we face in our relationships, such as differences of opinion or conflict, teach us important lessons about patience, empathy, and problem-solving. Furthermore, relationships inspire us and motivate us to be better. Seeing how other people face their own challenges or achieve their goals can serve as an example and encourage us to try harder in our own lives.

It is important to recognize that not all relationships are healthy. Sometimes, we can find ourselves in relationships that are toxic or that do us more harm than good. These relationships can drain us emotionally, make us feel bad about ourselves, or even affect our mental and physical health. Identifying these relationships and taking steps to protect ourselves, whether by setting clear boundaries or, in some cases, walking away from the relationship, is critical to our well-being. Mutual respect and unconditional support are the foundations of any healthy relationship, and if these are absent, we may need to reevaluate the relationship.

Finally, it is essential to remember that relationships, like us, change and evolve over time. As we grow and our circumstances change, our relationships can change too. Some relationships may strengthen and deepen, while others may fade or transform into something different. Accepting these changes and adapting to them is part of the natural process of life. Keeping an open mind and being willing to work on our relationships, even when it's difficult, is key to maintaining meaningful and lasting connections.

In conclusion, the relationships and support we receive from others are essential to our overall well-being. Healthy relationships provide us with emotional support, a sense of belonging, and an opportunity to grow and develop as people. However, maintaining these relationships requires effort, communication and understanding. By cultivating connections based on mutual respect and unconditional support, we can create an environment where we can all thrive. Ultimately, our relationships with others enrich our lives and provide us with a source of joy and well-being that we could hardly find on our own.

Nature as Medicine

Nature has been, since time immemorial, an inexhaustible source of healing and well-being. Before modern medicines existed, people turned to plants, fresh air, pure water, and the sun to heal their bodies and revitalize their minds. Today, although we live in a highly urbanized and technologically advanced world, nature remains one of the best medicines we have at our disposal. Connecting with the natural environment not only benefits our physical health, but also our mental and emotional health. This chapter explores how nature acts as a powerful medicine, and how we can harness its benefits to nourish our well-being in daily life.

The simple act of being outdoors, surrounded by trees, mountains, rivers or the sea, has an immediate positive effect on our body and mind. Numerous studies have shown that spending time in nature reduces stress and anxiety levels, lowers blood pressure, and improves immune system function. These benefits are due in part to nature's ability to reduce the production of the stress hormone cortisol. When we get away from the hustle and bustle of the city and immerse ourselves in a natural environment, our body enters a state of relaxation, allowing our nervous system to calm and our stress levels to decrease.

Nature also has a profound impact on our mental health. Spending time outdoors, whether walking in a park, hiking in the mountains, or simply sitting under a tree, helps us clear our minds and reduce negative thoughts. Contact with nature gives us a feeling of peace and tranquility that is difficult to find in other places. This connection with the natural environment allows us to disconnect from daily worries and reconnect with ourselves. Nature acts as a balm for the mind, helping us see things more clearly and find solutions to the problems we face.

In addition to its calming effects, nature also provides us with a dose of renewing energy. The fresh air, the sunlight, and the sound of running water or the singing of birds fill us with vitality and help us recharge our energies. This is especially important in a world where we often feel exhausted by the demands of work, traffic, and daily responsibilities. Spending time in nature gives us a break from all this and allows us to recharge our batteries, so we can face the day with more enthusiasm and positivity.

Nature not only offers us a place to relax and rejuvenate, but it also provides us with an endless source of inspiration and creativity. Natural landscapes, with their colors, shapes and sounds, stimulate our senses and inspire us to think more creatively. Many artists, writers and thinkers throughout history have found in nature an inexhaustible muse for their work. This inspiring effect is not just limited to artists; Anyone can benefit from the inspiration that nature offers. Simply being outdoors, observing the beauty around us, can open our minds to new ideas and perspectives.

Another important aspect of nature is its ability to connect us with something bigger than ourselves. When we find ourselves in the middle of a forest, facing an immense ocean, or contemplating a majestic mountain, it is difficult not to feel a deep sense of awe and humility. Nature reminds us how small we are compared to the vastness of the natural world, and at the same time, shows us that we are part of a larger whole. This connection with nature can give us a sense of purpose and belonging, helping us feel more at peace with ourselves and the world around us.

In addition to individual benefits, nature also plays a crucial role in building stronger, healthier communities. Activities like group hiking, community gardening, or beach cleanups not only connect us with nature, but they also connect us with other people. These activities foster a sense of community and allow us to share meaningful experiences with others. Teamwork and collaboration in a natural environment can strengthen the bonds between people and create a sense of unity and solidarity.

It is important to note that we do not need to live in the countryside or have access to large natural areas to enjoy the benefits that nature offers. Even in cities, we can find ways to connect with nature. Visiting parks, botanical gardens, or simply taking care of plants at home are effective ways to integrate nature into our daily lives. The key is to make a conscious effort to spend time outdoors and surround ourselves with natural elements, even in small doses. These moments, although brief, can have a significant impact on our overall well-being.

On the other hand, nature also teaches us valuable life lessons. By observing natural cycles, such as the change of seasons, the growth of plants, or the behavior of animals, we can learn about patience, adaptability, and the importance of living in harmony with our environment. Nature shows us that everything in life has its rhythm and that it is important to respect those rhythms, both in our environment and in ourselves. By learning from nature, we can apply these lessons to our daily lives, helping us live in a more balanced and conscious way.

In short, nature is a powerful medicine that is available to everyone. It offers us a refuge from stress and anxiety, fills us with energy and vitality, inspires us and connects us with something bigger than ourselves. By making a conscious effort to spend time outdoors and surrounding ourselves with natural beauty, we can significantly improve our physical, mental, and emotional health. Nature not only heals us, but also teaches us valuable lessons about life, growth and harmony. In an increasingly fast-paced and disconnected world, reconnecting with nature is more important than ever for our overall well-being.

The Magic of Silence

Silence, in a world full of noise and distractions, is an increasingly scarce and, at the same time, more valuable commodity. We live in a society that constantly bombards us with information, sounds, and visual stimuli, from the moment we wake up until we go to sleep. We rarely find a moment of true stillness, a moment to simply be, uninterrupted by the buzzing of phones, traffic, or the incessant hum of conversation. However, silence has a transformative power. It offers us a unique opportunity to reconnect with ourselves, reflect on our lives, and find an inner peace that is difficult to achieve in the midst of everyday hustle and bustle. This chapter explores the magic of silence and how we can incorporate it into our daily lives to improve our overall well-being.

Silence is not simply the absence of noise; It is a space where we can find ourselves in a way that is not possible anywhere else. In silence, our minds have the opportunity to rest and recharge. Often, we are so busy with our daily tasks and so immersed in constant noise that we don't realize how much we need a moment of stillness. Silence allows us to take a breath, stop, and listen to what is really happening inside of us. It is in these moments of silence when we can reflect on our emotions, our decisions, and the direction we are taking in life.

One of the most important benefits of silence is its ability to reduce stress. When we are in a quiet environment, our nervous system calms, and our levels of cortisol, the stress hormone, decrease. Silence acts as a natural antidote to the noise and pressures of modern life, helping us find mental and emotional balance. Even just a few minutes of silence a day can have a significant impact on our mental health. The simple act of sitting quietly, without distractions, can be incredibly relaxing and restorative.

In addition to its calming effects, silence also gives us mental clarity. In a world where we are constantly bombarded with information, it is easy to feel overwhelmed and confused. Silence allows us to organize our thoughts, prioritize what is really important, and make more conscious decisions. Instead of reacting impulsively to situations, silence gives us the space to reflect and respond in a more considered and balanced way. This mental clarity not only helps us make better decisions, but also allows us to live more intentionally and aligned with our values.

Silence is also a powerful means for introspection and self-knowledge. In stillness, we can explore our deepest emotions, our aspirations, and our concerns. We can ask important questions about who we are, what we want in life, and how we can grow and evolve as people. The introspection that silence facilitates helps us know ourselves better and understand our motivations, fears, and desires. This inner knowing is essential for our personal growth and allows us to live more authentically and meaningfully.

Another important aspect of silence is its ability to improve our relationships with others. In communication, silence is often underestimated, but it is a powerful tool. Listening silently when another person is speaking shows respect, empathy, and understanding. It allows us to capture not only the words, but also the tone, emotion, and nuances that are present in the conversation. Silence in communication also gives us time to think before responding, which can lead to more thoughtful and meaningful exchanges. By practicing silence in our interactions, we can build stronger, more genuine relationships.

Silence also plays a crucial role in creativity. Many artists, writers, and thinkers find that their best work emerges in moments of silence. Stillness allows our minds to wander, often leading to the generation of new ideas and perspectives. In silence, our minds are free to explore without the limitations of noise and distractions. This not only encourages creativity, but also allows us to solve problems more effectively. When we give ourselves permission to be silent, we allow inspiration to flow naturally and effortlessly.

For many, silence may seem uncomfortable at first. We are so used to constant noise that silence can feel strange, even disturbing. However, over time, we can learn to appreciate and value these moments of stillness. Practicing silence is a skill that can be developed, and the more we do it, the more benefits we experience. Starting with small moments of silence each day, such as during a walk, when you wake up, or before bed, can be a good starting point. Over time, these moments can extend and become an integral part of our daily routine.

It is important to remember that silence is not only an absence of external noise, but also a state of mind. Sometimes, even in a noisy environment, we can find a space of inner silence. This inner silence is the ability to remain calm and centered in the midst of chaos. Cultivating this inner silence through practices such as meditation or conscious breathing helps us remain calm and clear, no matter what is happening around us. This state of internal silence is an inexhaustible source of peace and stability, which allows us to face life with more serenity and strength.

In conclusion, silence is a powerful tool to improve our general well-being. It offers us an opportunity to reduce stress, find mental clarity, get to know ourselves better, and strengthen our relationships. Additionally, silence fosters creativity and helps us live more intentionally and meaningfully. In a world where noise and distractions are the norm, silence is a luxury we should all allow ourselves. By incorporating moments of silence into our daily lives, we can experience a profound transformation in how we feel, think, and live. Silence, in its simplicity, has a magic that can enrich our lives in ways we never imagined.

Creating Positive Routines

Creating positive routines is one of the most effective ways to improve our quality of life and general well-being. Routines, those habits that we repeat day after day, are the pillars on which we build our lives. From the moment we wake up until we go to sleep, our daily actions define who we are and how we feel. Therefore, establishing routines that support and nourish us is essential to live healthier, more productive and happier. This chapter explores the importance of creating positive routines, how to do it effectively, and the benefits they can bring to our daily lives.

The power of a well-established routine lies in its ability to automate healthy behaviors, freeing up mental space for other, more meaningful activities. When we incorporate positive practices into our daily routine, such as exercise, healthy eating, or meditation, these actions become second nature. We no longer need to spend mental energy deciding whether we should do them or not; They simply become part of our life. This automation allows us to be more consistent in our efforts toward wellness and helps us stay on track, even when we face challenges or moments of stress.

One of the first steps to creating a positive routine is to identify which areas of our lives we want to improve. This can include physical aspects, such as our health and fitness, or mental and emotional aspects, such as our inner peace or happiness. By having clarity about our goals, we can design routines that are aligned with what we really want to achieve. For example, if we want to improve our physical health, we can establish a morning exercise routine and opt for a balanced diet. If our goal is to reduce stress, we can incorporate daily practices such as meditation, deep breathing, or journal writing.

Once we have identified our goals, it is important to start gradually. Often, when we try to introduce too many changes at once, we feel overwhelmed and are more likely to abandon our efforts. Therefore, it is advisable to start with small adjustments that are manageable and sustainable. For example, if we want to adopt an exercise routine, we can start with short sessions of 10 or 15 minutes a day, and then gradually increase the duration and intensity. The same applies to other habits, such as healthy eating or meditation; Small consistent steps are more effective in the long term than large temporary changes.

Another key to creating positive routines is consistency. Routines work best when they are repeated at the same time every day, as this helps our brain associate certain times of the day with certain activities. For example, if we decide to exercise every morning when we wake up, over time our body and mind will get used to this practice and it will be easier to maintain it. Consistency also helps us create a sense of structure and order in our lives, which can be very beneficial for our emotional well-being. Knowing what comes next in our day gives us a feeling of control and security, which reduces anxiety and stress.

However, creating a positive routine doesn't mean we have to be rigid or inflexible. Life is unpredictable, and sometimes our circumstances change, which may require adjustments to our routines. It's important to be flexible and willing to adapt our routines as needed, without feeling guilty or frustrated. The key is to keep an open mind and remember that routines are here to support us, not limit us. If at any point we can't follow a routine as planned, we can make small adjustments and continue without missing a beat.

In addition to the physical and mental benefits, positive routines can also improve our relationships with others. When we establish habits that promote self-care, such as exercise, healthy eating, and stress management, we feel better about ourselves and this is reflected in the way we interact with others. We can also create routines that include quality time with our loved ones, such as family dinners, walks outdoors, or recreational activities. These practices strengthen family and friendly ties, and allow us to enjoy healthier and more satisfying relationships.

Another important aspect of routines is their ability to increase our productivity. When we organize our day around positive habits, we are better able to use our time efficiently. For example, by establishing a morning routine that includes exercise, a healthy breakfast, and a clear to-do list, we start the day with energy and focus, allowing us to be more productive in our daily activities. Routines also help us avoid procrastination, since by following a regular schedule, we reduce distractions and stay focused on our goals.

It is important to mention that creating positive routines is not only about including new activities, but also about eliminating or reducing those that do not benefit us. Identifying negative habits, such as spending too much time on social media, overeating, or avoiding exercise, is a crucial step to improving our lives. Replacing these habits with healthier alternatives, such as reading a book, cooking a nutritious meal, or practicing yoga, allows us to transform our routines in meaningful and lasting ways.

Creating positive routines can also be an act of self-compassion. We often feel pressured to do everything perfect, but the reality is that no one is perfect. Routines are not designed to be followed impeccably every day; They are meant to guide and support us on our path to a fuller and more satisfying life. It's important to be kind to ourselves when things don't go as planned. Accepting that there will be days when we won't be able to follow our routine to the letter and learning not to beat ourselves up about it is a crucial part of the process.

Finally, positive routines can be a source of satisfaction and happiness. When we see the progress we have made thanks to our routines, we feel a sense of accomplishment and pride. These small daily victories add up over time, leading to a more balanced and rewarding life. Routines also give us something to look forward to each day, whether it's a cup of tea in the morning, a walk in the park, or a conversation with a loved one at the end of the day. These small daily joys are what truly enrich our lives and allow us to enjoy the beauty of routine.

In conclusion, creating positive routines is a powerful way to improve our overall well-being. By establishing habits that support us physically, mentally, and emotionally, we can live healthier, more productive, and happier lives. Routines help us automate healthy behaviors, maintain consistency in our efforts, and enjoy greater clarity and focus in our lives. By being flexible, eliminating negative habits, and practicing self-compassion, we can make our routines a source of satisfaction and happiness. Over time, these routines become an integral part of our daily lives, guiding us toward a fuller and more meaningful existence.

Gratitude as a Lifestyle

Gratitude is one of the most powerful and transformative emotions we can experience. Although often considered simply an occasional act of saying thank you, gratitude has the potential to become a lifestyle, a way of seeing and experiencing the world that can enrich every aspect of our existence. Adopting gratitude as a lifestyle means cultivating an attitude of continuous appreciation, recognizing and valuing the blessings, large and small, that we encounter in our daily lives. This chapter explores how gratitude can transform our lives, how we can practice it consciously, and the benefits it can bring us both emotionally and physically.

Living with gratitude is not about ignoring the difficulties or challenges we face, but rather about consciously choosing to focus on the positive, even in the midst of adversity. We all go through difficult times, but gratitude helps us see beyond the immediate circumstances and find something to be grateful for. It can be something as simple as having a roof over our heads, the support of a loved one, or the beauty of a sunrise. This perspective not only allows us to face challenges with more resilience, but also helps us maintain a positive attitude, which is crucial for our overall well-being.

One of the first steps to adopting gratitude as a lifestyle is learning to recognize the things we can be grateful for. This may seem simple, but we are often so busy and caught up in the daily routine that we don't stop to appreciate what we have. A helpful practice to develop this skill is to keep a gratitude journal. At the end of each day, taking a few minutes to write down three things we are grateful for can have a profound impact on our perspective. These don't have to be big things; They can be small gestures, like a smile, a delicious meal, or a moment of peace. Over time, this practice trains us to look for the positive in our lives, which in turn makes us more aware and appreciative of our daily blessings.

Another important aspect of living with gratitude is expressing our gratitude to others. We often feel gratitude for the people around us, but we don't always express it. Saying "thank you" is a powerful act that not only strengthens our relationships, but also makes us feel more connected and supported. Whether it's a friend, family member, co-worker, or even a stranger who provided help in a time of need, expressing our gratitude creates a cycle of positivity and strengthens the bonds between people. Additionally, when we make a conscious effort to express our gratitude, we realize how many people contribute to our well-being, which makes us feel more supported and less alone.

Gratitude also has a significant impact on our physical health. Numerous studies have shown that people who practice gratitude regularly have better overall health. They have fewer blood pressure problems, sleep better, and experience fewer symptoms of stress-related illnesses. Gratitude helps us reduce stress because it allows us to focus on the positive, which in turn reduces the levels of cortisol, the stress hormone, in our body. Additionally, gratitude promotes a positive feedback loop, where feeling good leads us to be more grateful, which makes us feel even better.

Gratitude also plays a crucial role in our mental health. By shifting our focus toward what we have rather than what we lack, we can reduce feelings of anxiety, depression, and hopelessness. Gratitude helps us avoid the trap of comparison, which often leaves us feeling dissatisfied or inferior to others. Instead of comparing our lives to those of others, gratitude teaches us to value our own life as it is, with all its imperfections and challenges. This change in perspective allows us to enjoy the present more and experience greater satisfaction with life.

A key element to living with gratitude is the practice of mindfulness. Gratitude and mindfulness are closely related, as they both require us to be present and aware in the moment. When we are mindful, we are better able to notice and appreciate the things around us, from the warmth of the sun on our skin to the taste of our food. Mindfulness helps us disconnect from the autopilot we often live on and allows us to experience the world with greater depth and meaning. By combining mindfulness with gratitude, we can transform even the most routine activities into moments of appreciation and joy.

Gratitude can also be a source of strength in times of difficulty. When we face challenges, gratitude helps us maintain a balanced perspective, reminding us that even in the darkest moments, there are things we can be grateful for. This approach does not minimize our struggles, but it gives us the resilience needed to move forward. For example, during an illness, we can be grateful for the support of our loved ones, for access to medical care, or for small moments of relief. Gratitude in difficult times acts as an anchor that keeps us connected to the positive, preventing us from sinking into discouragement.

Furthermore, living with gratitude also has a contagious effect. When we practice gratitude, we inspire others to do the same. Our grateful attitude can influence the people around us, creating a more positive and harmonious environment in our communities. This ripple effect of gratitude can lead to a culture of appreciation and generosity, where people feel more valued and willing to help others. In this sense, gratitude not only improves our personal life, but also contributes to the well-being of those around us.

Incorporating gratitude into our daily lives also allows us to enjoy simple things more. Often, we are so focused on our long-term goals that we forget to appreciate the small joys we find along the way. Gratitude helps us stop and savor those moments, like a conversation with a friend, the aroma of coffee in the morning, or the sound of rain on the roof. These small pleasures are what truly enrich our lives and give us a feeling of fulfillment and satisfaction. By practicing gratitude, we learn to enjoy these moments more and live more fully.

Finally, gratitude helps us maintain an attitude of abundance. Instead of focusing on what we don't have, gratitude teaches us to value what we already have. This attitude of abundance makes us feel more satisfied with our lives and less driven by the desire to have more. By cultivating gratitude, we can free ourselves from the cycle of unfulfilled desire that often leads us to feel unhappy and envious. Instead, gratitude allows us to see the abundance in our lives for what it is, and gives us the peace and joy that comes from knowing that we already have enough.

In conclusion, adopting gratitude as a lifestyle has the power to transform our existence in a profound and meaningful way. By learning to recognize and appreciate the blessings in our daily lives, we can experience greater happiness, well-being, and satisfaction. Gratitude helps us maintain a positive outlook, reduce stress, and enjoy simple things more. Additionally, gratitude strengthens our relationships, improves our physical and mental health, and gives us the resilience needed to face life's challenges. By living with gratitude, we can find a constant source of joy and peace, and create a more fulfilling and meaningful life.

Simplify to Live Better

Simplifying our lives is a powerful way to improve our well-being and find more satisfaction in our daily lives. We live in a society that often pushes us to do more, have more, and want more, which can lead us to feel overwhelmed and disconnected from what really matters. However, when we choose to simplify, we are taking a conscious step to eliminate the noise, reduce stress, and focus on what is truly essential. This chapter explores how simplifying can transform our lives, how we can apply this approach in different areas, and the benefits of living in a simpler and more meaningful way.

Simplifying does not necessarily mean giving up the things we like or that are important to us. Rather, it's about making room for what we truly value by getting rid of the unnecessary. This can include material possessions, social commitments, or even thoughts and worries that weigh us down. By simplifying, we can free ourselves from unnecessary burdens and focus on what truly makes us happy and gives us meaning. This simplification process allows us to live with greater clarity and purpose, and helps us create a more balanced and rewarding life.

One of the most obvious areas where we can begin to simplify is in our physical environment. Many people find that having too much stuff can be a source of stress and anxiety. Clutter in our home or workplace can make us feel overwhelmed and distracted, hindering our ability to focus and relax. Simplifying our physical space means getting rid of objects that we no longer need or that do not bring us joy, and keeping only what we really use or value. This decluttering process, or clutter reduction, can be very liberating, as it allows us to create a more orderly, calm and pleasant environment.

The simplification process can also be applied to how we manage our time. We often feel pressured to fill every moment of our schedule with activities and commitments, which can lead us to feel exhausted and without time for ourselves. Simplifying our schedule means being more selective with how we choose to spend our time, prioritizing the activities that really matter to us and eliminating those that don't add value to us. This may include learning to say "no" to certain commitments, delegating tasks, or simply setting aside time to rest and recharge. By simplifying our schedule, we can reduce stress and enjoy a more balanced and satisfying life.

Another important aspect of simplifying our lives is learning to reduce mental noise. Our minds are constantly busy with thoughts, worries, and distractions, which can hinder our ability to relax and enjoy the present moment. Simplifying our thoughts involves being aware of what we allow into our minds and consciously choosing to focus on the positive. This can include practices such as meditation, mindfulness, or simply taking a moment to breathe deeply and clear our minds. By reducing mental noise, we can experience greater inner peace and clarity, allowing us to make better decisions and live more peacefully.

Relationships can also benefit from a simplified approach. Often, we surround ourselves with relationships that can be complicated or that do not provide us with the support we need. Simplifying our relationships means focusing on the people we truly value and share a meaningful connection with. This doesn't necessarily mean cutting ties with everyone else, but it does mean being more mindful of how we choose to invest our time and energy in our relationships. By focusing on relationships that bring us happiness and support, we can strengthen our ties with others and enjoy healthier, more satisfying relationships.

Conscious consumption is another important way to simplify our lives. Instead of hoarding things out of impulse or habit, we can opt for a more conscious and deliberate approach to our purchasing decisions. This involves thinking before buying, asking ourselves if we really need a product, and considering its impact on our lives and the environment. By consuming more consciously, we not only reduce the clutter in our lives, but also adopt a more sustainable and ethical lifestyle. This approach allows us to live with less, but with more meaning, since everything we own has a clear purpose and adds value to our lives.

Simplifying can also be applied to our finances. Our financial lives can often be a source of stress, especially when we find ourselves trapped in the cycle of overspending and debt. Simplifying our finances means taking a more conscious and responsible approach to how we manage our money. This can include creating a clear budget, reducing unnecessary expenses, and focusing on saving and investing in what really matters. By simplifying our finances, we can free up resources for the things we really value and reduce money anxiety.

Another area where simplifying can have a big impact is in our diet and lifestyle. We often feel pressured to follow complicated diets or intense exercise routines that can be difficult to maintain long-term. Simplifying our diet and exercise means opting for a more natural and balanced approach. This can include eating fresh, unprocessed foods, and choosing forms of exercise that we really enjoy and that fit into our lifestyle. By simplifying our diet and exercise routine, we can improve our health and well-being without feeling overwhelmed by the pressure of meeting unattainable standards.

Work is also an area where simplification can be beneficial. Many times, we find ourselves stuck in work routines that can be stressful or unsatisfying. Simplifying our work may involve reviewing our priorities, delegating tasks when possible, and looking for more efficient ways of doing things. It can also mean setting clear boundaries between work and personal life, to ensure we're not sacrificing our health or happiness on the altar of professional success. By simplifying our approach to work, we can reduce stress and find greater balance between our work and personal lives.

Technology is another area where simplification can be extremely useful. We live in an era where we are constantly connected, and although technology offers us many advantages, it can also be a source of distraction and stress. Simplifying our use of technology means being more aware of how and when we use it. This may include reducing the time we spend on social networks, limiting the notifications we receive, and creating technology-free spaces in our daily lives. By simplifying our relationship with technology, we can be more present in our lives, improve our relationships, and reduce information overload.

Simplifying also involves learning to let go. Often, we cling to things, ideas, or expectations that no longer serve us or even harm us. Learning to let go means accepting that we do not need to carry with us all the weight of the past or all the expectations for the future. Letting go is not about giving up, but about freeing ourselves from that which does not allow us to move forward or that prevents us from enjoying the present. By simplifying our emotional life, we can free ourselves from resentments, fears, and unrealistic expectations, allowing ourselves to live in a lighter and more joyful way.

Ultimately, simplifying to live better is an act of self-care and self-love. By making conscious decisions about what we allow into our lives, we are saying "yes" to what really matters and "no" to what drains us or distances us from our values and goals. Simplifying allows us to live with more intention, aligned with our true desires and needs, and helps us create a life that is an authentic reflection of who we are and what we value. It's not about living with less, but about living with more meaning and purpose.

In conclusion, simplifying our lives can have a profound impact on our well-being and happiness. By reducing clutter, managing our time better, and focusing on what is essential, we can live in a more balanced, calm, and satisfying way. Simplifying allows us to free up space for what really matters, whether in our relationships, finances, work, or simply our peace of mind. By adopting simplicity as an approach to life, we can find more joy in the everyday, reduce stress, and live with greater clarity and purpose. Living more simply does not mean giving up what we love, but rather making space for what truly nourishes us and makes us happy.

The Power of Breath

Breathing is one of the most basic and essential functions of our body, but we often overlook it. Breathing is something we do automatically, without even thinking about it, and yet it is a powerful tool we have at our disposal to improve our physical, mental and emotional well-being. The power of the breath lies in its ability to influence how we feel, how we react to stress, and how we connect with ourselves in the present moment. In this chapter, we will explore how breathing can be a transformative tool for our health and how we can learn to use it consciously to live in a more balanced and fulfilling way.

Breathing is the direct connection between our body and our mind. When we breathe consciously, we can influence our emotional state, calm our mind, and relax our body. This is because breathing is closely linked to the autonomic nervous system, which controls our responses to stress. When we are stressed or anxious, our breathing tends to become rapid and shallow, which in turn sends signals to our brain that we are in danger. However, by taking conscious control of our breathing and making it slower and deeper, we can activate our body's relaxation response, slowing our heart rate, reducing blood pressure, and promoting a state of calm.

One of the simplest and most effective breathing techniques we can use is diaphragmatic breathing, also known as abdominal breathing. This technique involves inhaling deeply through the nose, allowing air to fill our lungs and causing our abdomen to expand. Then, we exhale slowly through the mouth, letting the abdomen return to its original position. Practicing diaphragmatic breathing allows us to fully use our lungs, improving the body's oxygenation and helping us release accumulated tension. Additionally, this type of breathing anchors us in the present moment, reducing the scattered mind and bringing us back to the here and now.

Another powerful technique is mindful breathing, which is simply paying attention to each inhalation and exhalation. We can do it at any time of the day, while we walk, work or even when we are resting. Conscious breathing helps us be more present and cultivate an attitude of mindfulness. When we focus on our breathing, we stop worrying about the past or anticipating the future, and begin to experience the present with greater clarity. This simple act of observing our breathing can have a calming effect, helping us reduce stress and improve our mood.

Breathing also plays a crucial role in stress management. In stressful situations, it is common for our breathing to become rapid and shallow, which can increase symptoms of anxiety and tension. However, we can counteract this automatic response by practicing slow, controlled breathing. A useful technique is box breathing, which involves inhaling for four seconds, holding your breath for four seconds, exhaling for four seconds, and then holding your lungs empty for four seconds before repeating the cycle. This technique not only calms the nervous system, but also gives us a greater sense of control over our emotions, allowing us to respond to stressful situations in a more calm and effective way.

Breathing can also be a powerful tool to improve our physical health. Breathing deeply and regularly improves blood circulation, which helps deliver oxygen and nutrients to all the cells in the body. Additionally, good breathing strengthens the immune system by increasing the amount of oxygen available to immune cells, helping them better fight infections. Deep breathing also promotes the elimination of toxins through the lymphatic system, which contributes to better detoxification of the body and greater overall vitality.

Regularly practicing breathing exercises can also help us improve the quality of sleep. Many people experience insomnia or difficulty sleeping due to a agitated mind or accumulated stress. By practicing breathing techniques before bed, we can calm the nervous system, reduce mental activity, and prepare the body for more restful sleep. Deep, slow breathing, combined with an attitude of relaxation, can be an effective way to fall asleep more quickly and improve the quality of your night's rest.

In addition to its physical and mental benefits, breathing also has an impact on our spiritual and emotional lives. In many spiritual traditions, breathing is seen as a way to connect with the divine or our inner essence. Conscious breathing allows us to enter a state of meditation and heightened awareness, helping us connect with our true nature and experience a sense of peace and unity. Breathing can be a gateway to greater self-knowledge and a greater connection with the world around us.

Breathing can also help us release repressed emotions. Often, emotions that we have not expressed or processed properly remain trapped in our body, manifesting as physical tension or emotional discomfort. By practicing conscious breathing, we can release these emotions and allow our energy to flow more freely. For example, during a deep breathing session, we may notice a particular emotion arising, such as sadness or anger. Instead of repressing it, we can allow that emotion to be expressed through our breathing, releasing it and making room for feelings of peace and well-being.

Breathing is also a powerful tool to improve our concentration and focus. In a world full of distractions, staying focused can be a challenge. However, by practicing conscious breathing, we can train our mind to stay focused on the task at hand. When we feel our mind starting to wander, we can use our breath as an anchor to bring it back to the present. By doing this repeatedly, we develop a greater ability to concentrate, allowing us to be more productive and present in our daily activities.

Additionally, breathing can be a form of daily self-care. In the midst of our busy lives, we often forget to take a moment for ourselves. However, simply taking a few minutes each day to breathe consciously can be a way to reconnect with our body and mind, and take care of our well-being. These moments of conscious breathing don't have to be long or complicated; They can be as simple as taking three deep breaths before starting the day, or taking a break during a busy day. These small moments of self-care can have a big impact on our overall well-being.

Breathing also teaches us the importance of patience and acceptance. When we practice conscious breathing, we learn to be patient with ourselves and the process. It is not always easy to stay focused or calm the mind, and we may encounter resistance or challenges. However, by continuing to breathe with awareness, we learn to accept the moment as it is, without judging it or trying to change it. This attitude of acceptance allows us to live more peacefully and be kinder to ourselves.

Finally, breathing is a reminder of our connection to life. Every breath we take is a reminder that we are alive and that life flows through us. By honoring our breath, we honor life itself. Breathing connects us with nature, with others and with the universe as a whole. It is a life force that sustains and nourishes us, and by learning to breathe consciously, we can live more fully, more consciously, and more in harmony with the world around us.

In conclusion, breathing is a simple but powerful tool that we have at our disposal at all times. By learning to breathe consciously, we can improve our physical, mental and emotional health, reduce stress, and live more balanced and full lives. Breathing connects us with the present moment, helps us release tensions and emotions, and allows us to live with greater peace and clarity. By incorporating conscious breathing into our daily lives, we can transform our experience of life, creating a calmer, more fulfilling and vital existence.

Mental Health and Balance

Mental health is an essential component of our overall well-being, and finding balance in our lives is essential to maintaining it. We live in a world full of challenges and responsibilities that can affect our mental state, causing stress, anxiety, and exhaustion. However, taking care of our mental health is not just a matter of avoiding stress; It is a continuous process of self-awareness, self-care, and developing skills to handle life's ups and downs. In this chapter, we will explore how we can nourish our mental health and achieve balance in our daily lives to live more fully and consciously.

Mental health begins with self-acceptance. Accepting ourselves as we are, with our strengths and weaknesses, is the first step towards a healthy mind. We often set impossible standards for ourselves or compare ourselves to others, which can lead to feelings of inadequacy or low self-esteem. Learning to accept our imperfections and value ourselves for who we are rather than what we do is crucial to maintaining a balanced mind. This self-acceptance does not mean settling for our limitations, but rather recognizing them and working on them with compassion and patience.

Another key to good mental health is proper stress management. Stress is a natural response to life's demands, but when it becomes chronic, it can have negative effects on our well-being. It is important to learn to identify the sources of stress in our lives and develop strategies to manage it. This can include relaxation techniques such as meditation, conscious breathing or yoga, as well as practicing activities that help us disconnect and recharge, such as spending time in nature, reading a good book or enjoying a hobby. Setting clear boundaries on our responsibilities and learning to say no when necessary are also effective ways to reduce stress and protect our mental health.

Work-life balance is another essential aspect of maintaining mental health. In a world where the lines between work and free time have blurred, it's easy to fall into the trap of always being available or taking work worries home. However, to keep our minds healthy, it is vital to create a clear space between work and our personal lives. This may involve setting defined work schedules, disconnecting from electronic devices during off-duty hours, and making sure we spend quality time on our relationships and activities that bring us joy and satisfaction.

Interpersonal relationships play a crucial role in our mental health. We are social beings by nature, and our interactions with others have a significant impact on how we feel. Having positive, supportive relationships helps us feel connected, understood, and valued. On the other hand, toxic or conflictive relationships can drain our energy and negatively affect our emotional state. It is important to surround ourselves with people who support us and push us to be our best version, and learn to establish healthy boundaries in those relationships that do not contribute to our well-being.

Managing emotions is another central aspect of mental health. We all experience a range of emotions throughout the day, from joy to sadness, anger or frustration. The important thing is not to avoid these emotions, but to learn to manage them in a healthy way. This involves recognizing our emotions without judging them, understanding where they come from and how they affect our behavior, and finding constructive ways to express them. For example, instead of repressing anger, we can learn to communicate our feelings assertively and respectfully. Likewise, instead of sinking into sadness, we can seek support or engage in activities that lift our spirits.

Self-care is essential to maintain mental balance. Taking care of our mind is as important as taking care of our body. This means giving ourselves permission to rest when we need it, making sure we are getting enough sleep, eating well, and exercising regularly. It also means spending time on activities that bring us joy and satisfaction, whether it's spending time with loved ones, practicing a hobby, or simply enjoying a quiet moment. Self-care is not selfish; It is a necessity to be able to function well in our lives and be able to care for others.

Mindset also plays a crucial role in our mental health. Adopting a growth mindset, rather than a fixed mindset, allows us to see challenges as opportunities to learn and grow rather than insurmountable obstacles. A growth mindset helps us stay resilient in the face of difficulties, be more adaptable, and see mistakes as part of the learning process. This mindset also encourages self-efficacy, that is, the belief in our ability to influence the events in our lives and achieve our goals.

Gratitude is another powerful tool for maintaining mental health. Practicing gratitude regularly helps us focus on the positive aspects of our lives, which in turn improves our mood and overall well-being. Gratitude reminds us that despite challenges, there is always something to be grateful for. Whether for health, the love of our loved ones, or small daily joys, cultivating an attitude of gratitude allows us to see life from a more positive and balanced perspective.

Connecting with nature can also have a profound impact on our mental health. Spending time outdoors, surrounded by nature, has calming and revitalizing effects. Nature offers us a space to disconnect from the noise and hustle and bustle of daily life, and to reconnect with what is essential. Whether it's taking a walk in the park, spending time on the beach, or simply watching the stars, nature helps us reduce stress, improve our mood, and feel more at peace with ourselves.

Finally, it is important to remember that mental health is not a static state, but rather a continuous process of adaptation and growth. There will be good days and bad days, moments of balance and moments of challenge. The important thing is to develop the tools and strategies necessary to navigate these ups and downs with resilience and compassion. By learning to take care of our minds, manage stress, cultivate healthy relationships, and practice self-care, we can build a solid foundation for our mental health and find a balance that allows us to live more fully and satisfyingly.

In short, mental health and balance are fundamental pillars for a healthy and happy life. Taking care of our mind is a process that requires attention, self-care, and the willingness to learn and grow. By adopting habits and practices that promote our mental health, we can live with greater balance, resilience and satisfaction, enjoying a fuller and more conscious life.

Anna Baker

The Value of Disconnection

In the digital age we live in, we are more connected than ever. Our lives are intertwined with technology, from smartphones to social media and online work platforms. This constant connectivity offers us many advantages, such as the ability to communicate instantly with people around the world, access information immediately, and perform tasks more efficiently. However, this hyperconnectivity also comes at a cost, and it's easy to forget the value that disconnection has for our mental health and overall well-being.

Disconnecting does not mean giving up technology completely, but rather finding a balance that allows us to enjoy its benefits without it negatively interfering with our lives. Disconnection is an act of self-care, an opportunity to recharge our energies, reflect and reconnect with ourselves and the real world around us. In this chapter, we will explore why it is so important to unplug and how we can do it effectively to improve our quality of life.

One of the main benefits of disconnection is the reduction of stress. The constant pressure to always be available and connected can be overwhelming. Incessant notifications, urgent emails, and the need to respond quickly to messages can create a sense of urgency and anxiety that affects our peace of mind. By disconnecting, we give ourselves a break from this constant demand on our attention. We allow ourselves to relax, reduce mental noise, and take a step back to see things more clearly. This rest is essential to avoid exhaustion and maintain a balanced state of mind.

Disconnection also allows us to reconnect with what really matters. When we're constantly distracted by our screens, it's easy to lose sight of our priorities and the meaningful relationships in our lives. By unplugging, we can spend quality time with our families, friends, and ourselves. This quality time strengthens our relationships, allows us to share authentic experiences and deepen our emotional connections. Additionally, by disconnecting, we also have the opportunity to reflect on our personal goals, desires, and needs, which helps us live more intentionally and consciously.

Another important aspect of disconnection is its positive impact on our creativity and productivity. We often think that being always connected makes us more productive, but the reality is that constant interruptions and distractions can decrease our ability to concentrate and be creative. The mind needs space to wander, to daydream, and to process ideas deeply. By disconnecting, we give our mind the space it needs to be creative, to find solutions to problems and to develop new ideas. It is in these moments of disconnection that our best ideas often emerge and we come up with innovative solutions to the challenges we face.

Disconnection is also essential for our physical health. Spending long hours in front of a screen can have negative effects on our body, such as vision problems, headaches and general fatigue. Additionally, the lack of physical activity associated with being glued to our screens can contribute to a sedentary lifestyle, which increases the risk of health problems such as obesity, heart disease, and musculoskeletal problems. By disconnecting, we give ourselves the opportunity to move more, be outdoors, and take better care of our bodies. Simple activities such as walking, exercising or simply being in nature have a positive impact on our physical and mental health.

Disconnection also allows us to practice full attention, or mindfulness, which is the ability to be present in the current moment without judging it. When we are constantly connected, our minds are divided between the here and now and the digital world. We find ourselves checking our phones during meals, while chatting with friends, or even when we're alone, preventing us from fully enjoying these experiences. By unplugging, we can practice mindfulness, savoring every moment, whether it's a conversation, a meal, or a walk. This not only enriches our experiences, but also reduces stress and helps us feel more satisfied with our lives.

Disconnection is also an opportunity to rediscover hobbies and activities that bring us joy. Instead of spending hours scrolling through social media or watching TV shows, we can spend that time doing activities we're truly passionate about. Reading a good book, painting, playing a musical instrument, cooking a special meal or playing a sport are examples of activities that are not only rewarding, but also allow us to express ourselves and develop our skills. By unplugging, we can rediscover these passions and find new ways to enjoy our free time.

It is important to remember that disconnection does not have to be radical or permanent. It is not about giving up technology completely, but about establishing healthy limits that allow us to enjoy its benefits without sacrificing our well-being. This may include setting specific times to check email, turning off notifications during rest hours, or dedicating certain hours of the day to screen-free activities. It can also be helpful to designate spaces in our home as technology-free zones, such as the bedroom, to ensure that we have a place where we can relax without digital distractions.

Disconnection also allows us to reconnect with nature, which is essential for our well-being. Spending time outdoors, breathing fresh air and feeling the breeze on our skin, has a revitalizing effect on our mind and body. Nature offers us an escape from the bustle and demands of modern life, providing us with a space for reflection, peace and connection with something bigger than ourselves. Whether it's a walk in the park, a hike in the mountains or simply sitting in a garden, these moments of disconnection in nature are essential to recharge our energies and restore our internal balance.

Disconnection also has a positive impact on our interpersonal relationships. When we are always connected to our devices, we run the risk of being emotionally disconnected from the people around us. It's easy to be tempted to check your phone during a conversation or prioritize online interactions over face-to-face interactions. However, human relationships require presence and attention to flourish. By disconnecting, we can be truly present with our loved ones, actively listening, sharing meaningful moments, and strengthening the bonds that unite us.

Additionally, disconnection gives us the opportunity to practice silence and solitude, which is crucial for our emotional and mental well-being. In a world full of noise and constant stimuli, silence can be a refuge that allows us to listen to our own thoughts, reflect on our experiences and find inner peace. Solitude, on the other hand, should not be seen as something negative, but as a valuable time to reconnect with ourselves, to know ourselves better and to recharge our energies. These moments of silence and solitude are essential to maintaining a balanced mind and a healthy emotional life.

Finally, it is important to remember that disconnection is an act of resistance in a world that values productivity and constant availability. Disconnecting is an act of personal affirmation, a reminder that our worth does not depend on our ability to always be available or to respond immediately to every message. It is an act of self-care and respect for ourselves, which allows us to prioritize our mental health, our relationships and our general well-being. By disconnecting, we reclaim our time and attention, and allow ourselves to live more fully and authentically.

In conclusion, the value of disconnection lies in its ability to improve our mental health, strengthen our relationships, stimulate our creativity and reconnect us with what really matters. Disconnecting does not mean giving up technology, but rather finding a balance that allows us to enjoy its benefits without sacrificing our well-being. By practicing disconnection regularly, we can reduce stress, live more mindfully, and enjoy a more balanced and satisfying life. In a world that constantly pushes us to stay connected, disconnection is a powerful act of self-care and an essential tool for living more consciously and fully.

Feeding Creativity

Creativity is one of the most valuable and fascinating qualities of the human being. It is the spark that ignites innovation, problem solving and artistic expression. Nurturing creativity is not only important for those working in artistic or innovative fields, but for all of us, as creativity enriches our lives, allows us to see the world from new perspectives and find unique solutions to everyday challenges. In this chapter, we will explore how we can nurture and cultivate our creativity on a daily basis, and why it is essential to living a fuller and more satisfying life.

Creativity is not a gift reserved for a select few; It is an innate ability that we all possess. However, like any other skill, creativity needs to be nurtured and practiced to flourish. We often fall into the trap of thinking that creativity is something that just happens, a flash of inspiration that arrives unexpectedly. While it is true that creative ideas sometimes arise spontaneously, it is also true that we can create the conditions for creativity to thrive in our lives.

A first step to nurturing creativity is to cultivate curiosity. Curiosity is the desire to explore, learn and discover new things. It is the engine that drives our mind to ask questions, seek answers and see the world with fresh eyes. When we allow ourselves to be curious, we open the door to new ideas and possibilities. We can nourish our curiosity by reading about unfamiliar topics, exploring new places, interacting with people from different backgrounds and cultures, or simply observing our surroundings carefully. Curiosity keeps us mentally active and helps us connect ideas in unexpected ways.

Another fundamental aspect to feed creativity is mental space. Creativity needs space to develop, both literally and figuratively. In a world full of distractions and obligations, it is easy to feel overwhelmed and with your mind occupied by an endless list of tasks. However, creativity flourishes in quiet moments, when our minds are free to wander and explore. Creating time in our day for reflection, meditation or simply to be silent is essential to allow creative ideas to emerge. This mental space can also include the practice of relaxing activities, such as walking, exercising or spending time in nature, which allow us to disconnect from external noise and connect with our inner world.

Creativity is also fueled by the diversity of experiences. Exposing ourselves to a variety of experiences, cultures and ways of thinking enriches our minds and provides us with a resource bank from which to draw ideas. Traveling, learning a new language, attending cultural events or simply trying something new, such as a hobby or sport, opens us to new perspectives and allows us to see things from different angles. This diversity of experiences not only broadens our horizon, but also helps us make connections between seemingly disparate ideas, which is key to creativity.

Another important factor in fueling creativity is the practice of divergent thinking. Divergent thinking is the ability to generate multiple solutions or ideas from a single starting point. Instead of looking for a single correct answer, divergent thinking invites us to explore all possibilities, even those that seem unusual or unconventional. We can practice divergent thinking through simple exercises, such as brainstorming, where we challenge ourselves to generate as many ideas as possible in a short period of time, without judging their quality or viability at that moment. This practice helps us free our minds from restrictions and open ourselves to new ways of thinking.

Creativity is also fueled by experimentation and play. Many times, creative ideas emerge when we allow ourselves to play with concepts and experiment with different approaches. Play frees us from the pressure of having to find the perfect solution and allows us to explore new possibilities without fear of failure. This playful attitude is essential for creativity, as it allows us to take risks and discover new things. Whether we're drawing, writing, cooking, or problem-solving, adopting a gaming mindset helps us keep an open mind and enjoy the creative process.

Resilience also plays a crucial role in creativity. Throughout the creative process, it is common to encounter obstacles, failures and blockages. These challenges can be daunting, but they are a natural part of the creative path. Resilience allows us to persist in our ideas and projects, even when things don't go as we expect. Learning to see failures as opportunities to learn and grow is essential to keeping creativity alive.

Resilience teaches us not to give up in the face of difficulties and to move forward, knowing that each failed attempt brings us one step closer to a successful idea or solution.

Collaboration is another element that can enrich our creativity. Working with others offers us the opportunity to combine our ideas with those of others, often resulting in more innovative and original solutions. Collaboration challenges us to step out of our comfort zones, consider different points of view, and find ways to integrate different ideas into a cohesive whole. Furthermore, by collaborating, we can learn new skills and techniques from others, which enriches our own creative capacity. Creativity, on many occasions, is the result of a collective effort, where ideas are built and evolve through interaction with others.

It is important to note that creativity is not always linear or predictable. Sometimes creative ideas can take time to develop, and we may experience periods of creative block. At these times, it is crucial to be patient and not force the process. Creativity takes time, and often the best ideas come when we least expect it. Instead of putting pressure on ourselves to find an immediate solution, we can take a break, change focus, or simply allow ideas to mature naturally. Patience and trust in the creative process are essential to keep the spark of creativity alive.

Furthermore, creativity is not limited to the arts or innovation; It is a skill that we can apply in all aspects of our lives. From finding new ways to organize our home to solving problems at work or improving our personal relationships, creativity allows us to address everyday challenges more effectively and satisfyingly. By adopting a creative mindset, we become more flexible, adaptable, and able to find solutions to the problems we face. Creativity helps us see the world with new eyes and find beauty and possibility in the most common situations.

Finally, it is important to remember that creativity is a continuous and constantly evolving process. Nurturing our creativity requires a daily commitment to curiosity, exploration and experimentation. By keeping our minds open, allowing ourselves to play, and being willing to learn from failures, we can cultivate a life rich in creativity. This creativity not only enriches our personal lives, but also allows us to contribute more meaningfully to the world around us.

In short, nurturing creativity is a practice that allows us to live more fully, innovatively and satisfyingly. Creativity opens us to new possibilities, helps us solve problems in unique ways, and allows us to express ourselves in ways that fill us with joy and purpose. By nurturing our curiosity, creating mental space, experimenting with new ideas, and collaborating with others, we can keep our creativity alive and vibrant. Creativity not only helps us face life's challenges with ingenuity and resilience, it also allows us to enjoy a richer existence, full of color, excitement and possibility.

The Joy of Slow Movement

In a world that seems to move at breakneck speed, where haste is the norm and efficiency is valued above all else, the simple act of moving slowly can seem almost subversive. However, there is deep joy and endless benefits in slow movement. This not only invites us to slow down and be more aware of our bodies and the environment around us, but also allows us to experience life in a richer and more meaningful way. In this chapter, we will explore the importance of slow movement, how it can transform our relationship with time and space, and how we can incorporate it into our lives to find greater well-being and inner peace.

Slow movement, in its essence, is an invitation to be present in each moment. Unlike the frenetic pace we are used to, slow movement asks us to slow down, to pay attention to every step, every breath, every gesture. When we move slowly, we give ourselves the gift of time. We can notice details that would otherwise go unnoticed: the soft rustle of leaves under our feet, the feel of the wind on our skin, the steady beat of our heart. Instead of rushing from one place to another, slow movement allows us to savor the journey, to fully experience each moment.

One of the biggest benefits of slow movement is its ability to reduce stress. We live in a society that rewards productivity and often equates a person's worth with how much they can accomplish in the shortest amount of time. This constant focus on speed and efficiency can lead us to feel anxious, exhausted, and disconnected from ourselves. Slow movement, on the other hand, offers us respite. It reminds us that it is not always necessary to rush, that it is okay to take things slowly, that there is nothing wrong with moving at a slower pace. By allowing ourselves to move slowly, we reduce the pressure we feel to meet external expectations and give ourselves permission to simply be.

Slow movement also encourages body awareness. In a world full of distractions, it's easy to disconnect from our bodies, ignore the signals they send us, or even misinterpret them. Fast movement can contribute to this disconnection, as it often leads us to act automatically, without giving much thought to what we are doing or how we are feeling. Slow movement, on the other hand, forces us to pay attention. When we move slowly, we can feel how our muscles tense and relax, how our balance changes with each step, how our breathing aligns with the rhythm of our body. This body awareness helps us become more in tune with our physical and emotional needs, and allows us to respond to them more effectively.

Additionally, slow movement can be a deeply meditative practice. By moving slowly, we can focus on the present in a way that is often difficult to achieve when we move fast. Each movement becomes an opportunity to practice mindfulness, to be completely immersed in what we are doing, without distractions or worries about the past or the future. Whether we are walking, doing yoga, cooking, or simply doing everyday tasks, slow movement allows us to transform these activities into a form of moving meditation. This mindfulness practice not only improves our mental and emotional health, but also helps us develop greater gratitude for life's little moments.

Slow movement can also improve our relationships with others. When we move quickly, it is easy to fall into the trap of superficiality, of interacting with others in a hurry and without paying them the attention they deserve. Slow movement invites us to be more conscious in our interactions, to take the time to really listen, to observe, to be present with the people around us. By slowing down, we can build deeper, more meaningful connections, based on mutual understanding and respect. The simple act of sitting together in silence, of walking side by side without rushing, of sharing a meal without the urge to finish it quickly, can strengthen our bonds with others and make us feel more connected and supported.

Incorporating slow movement into our lives doesn't mean we have to give up efficiency or productivity. In fact, many times, moving slowly allows us to be more effective, as it gives us the opportunity to reflect, plan carefully, and avoid mistakes that can arise from haste. Slow movement helps us find a balance, knowing when it's time to pick up the pace and when it's time to slow down. This balance is essential to maintain our energy and avoid burnout, and allows us to live more sustainably and rewardingly.

A clear example of the benefits of slow movement is found in practices such as tai chi and yoga, where each movement is performed with a clear intention and purpose. These disciplines teach us to be aware of each part of our body, to coordinate our movements with our breathing, and to find calm in the slow pace. Through these practices, we can learn to apply the principles of slow movement to other areas of our lives, from how we walk to how we work, interact with others, or simply how we relax.

It is also important to mention that slow movement does not only refer to physical movement. It can also apply to the way we think, feel and make decisions. Instead of rushing to conclusions, slow movement invites us to reflect, to consider different perspectives, to allow ourselves time to feel and process our emotions. This slower approach helps us make more conscious decisions aligned with our values and needs, and allows us to live in a way that feels more authentic and fulfilling.

Throughout history, many cultures have valued slow movement as a form of wisdom and balance. From the meditative walks of Buddhist monks to tea ceremonies in Japan, slow movement has been a way to connect with oneself, others, and the natural world. In our modern lives, reclaiming this tradition can be a powerful way to counteract the stress and alienation we often feel. The slow movement reminds us that life is not a race, but a journey that deserves to be enjoyed at every step.

Finally, it is important to remember that slow movement is not a one-size-fits-all solution, but it can be a valuable tool to improve our quality of life. It offers us a way to find peace and contentment in a world that often seems chaotic and fast-paced. It teaches us to value quality over quantity, to prioritize presence over speed, and to find joy in the small moments. By embracing slow movement, we can not only reduce stress and improve our health, but we can also discover greater joy and gratitude in our daily lives.

In short, the joy of slow movement lies in its ability to reconnect with ourselves, others, and the world around us. It is a practice that invites us to slow down, be more aware, and find beauty and meaning in everyday moments. Through slow movement, we can learn to live in a more full, balanced and satisfying way, and discover that the true richness of life is found in the details, in small gestures and in full presence in each moment.

Love Yourself

Loving yourself is one of the most important and transformative acts you can do in your life. It is a concept that is often misinterpreted as selfishness or vanity, but in reality, self-love is the foundation on which a full, balanced and meaningful life is built. Without genuine love for yourself, it is difficult to find inner peace, contentment, and healthy relationships. In this chapter, we will explore what it really means to love yourself, why it is essential to your well-being, and how you can cultivate this love in your daily life.

Loving yourself begins with unconditional acceptance of who you are right now. We often fall into the trap of thinking that we will only be worthy of love once we achieve certain goals or achieve an idealized version of ourselves. You may think that you will only deserve love when you lose weight, get a promotion at work, or overcome some personal weakness. However, true self-love has no conditions. It's not about loving yourself only when you think you are perfect, but about loving yourself precisely in the midst of your imperfections. It's about looking in the mirror and recognizing that you are enough just the way you are, with all your strengths and weaknesses, your achievements and failures.

One of the fundamental aspects of self-love is self-compassion. Self-compassion means treating yourself with the same kindness, understanding, and patience that you would offer a dear friend. Often, we are our harshest critics, berating ourselves for every mistake and judging ourselves harshly. This self-criticism can be devastating to our self-esteem and emotional well-being. Practicing self-compassion means learning to be gentler with ourselves, to forgive ourselves when we make mistakes, and to remember that we are all human, with flaws and limitations. Instead of beating yourself up for not being perfect, self-compassion invites you to support yourself through difficult times, speak to yourself with words of encouragement, and recognize that failure is a natural part of growth.

Self-love also means prioritizing your well-being. This means making decisions that benefit you in the long run, even if they aren't always the easiest or most popular. For example, it can mean saying "no" to commitments that drain you, setting healthy boundaries in your relationships, or making time to take care of yourself physically and emotionally. Prioritizing your well-being is not a selfish act, but a way to ensure you have the energy and resilience necessary to live a fulfilling life. When you love yourself, you understand that it is your responsibility to take care of yourself, because only when you are good with yourself can you offer the best of yourself to others.

Furthermore, loving yourself requires recognizing and honoring your needs and desires. We often feel guilty for having needs, especially if we believe that our needs are not as important as those of others. But ignoring or minimizing what you really need to be happy and healthy only leads to dissatisfaction and resentment. Honoring your needs means listening to yourself, understanding what is essential to your well-being, and taking steps to meet those needs. It can be as simple as taking time each day to do something you enjoy, making sure your relationships are reciprocal and fulfilling, or seeking help when you need it.

Self-love also involves working on accepting your body. We live in a society that often sends us conflicting and unrealistic messages about what our bodies should be like. These messages can lead us to feel dissatisfied with our appearance and constantly strive to achieve an unattainable ideal. However, loving yourself means accepting your body as it is, with its curves, its wrinkles, its scars, and everything that makes it unique. It is learning to see your body not only as something that must meet certain aesthetic standards, but as the vehicle that allows you to experience life. Accepting your body means caring for it with love, feeding it well, moving it with joy and treating it with respect.

Another crucial facet of self-love is authenticity. Being authentic means being true to yourself, acting in accordance with your values and beliefs, and not trying to mold yourself to fit the expectations of others. Often, in an effort to be accepted or to be liked by others, we can lose sight of who we really are. However, loving yourself requires that you stay true to yourself, even when that means being different or not fitting into certain groups or social norms. Authenticity allows you to live a life that feels true and meaningful, because it is aligned with who you are at the core of your being.

Self-love is also closely related to self-esteem. Self-esteem is the assessment you have of yourself, and is based on the perception of your worth and your abilities. Loving yourself means cultivating a healthy self-esteem, based on a balanced recognition of your strengths and your areas for improvement. It is not about thinking that you are superior to others, but rather having a calm confidence in your inherent value as a person. Healthy self-esteem allows you to face challenges with more resilience, because you know that, no matter what, you have the internal tools to handle situations and move forward.

Loving yourself also means surrounding yourself with people who value and support you. Healthy relationships are a fundamental part of emotional well-being and self-love. If you surround yourself with people who respect you, who encourage you to be the best version of yourself, and who accept you for who you are, you are more likely to maintain a positive self-image. On the other hand, toxic relationships can undermine your self-esteem and make you feel unworthy of love. Loving yourself means being selective about the people you allow in your life and being willing to walk away from relationships that don't benefit you.

Finally, self-love is an ongoing process. It is not something that is achieved once and for all, but requires constant and conscious work. There will be days when you feel more connected to yourself and others when you will struggle to maintain that connection. The important thing is to remember that self-love is not linear and that it is normal to have ups and downs on this path. The essential thing is to keep moving forward, keep practicing self-compassion, keep prioritizing your well-being, and remember that you deserve love, simply because you exist.

In conclusion, loving yourself is the foundation on which a full and balanced life is built. It is an act of courage and commitment to yourself, which allows you to live with more peace, joy and authenticity. By learning to love yourself, you not only improve your relationship with yourself, but you also become more capable of loving and caring for others. This self-love is the key to a richer, more fulfilling life, and while the path may not always be easy, it is undoubtedly one of the most valuable journeys you can take.

Celebrating Life

Celebrating life is a deeply meaningful act that goes beyond holidays and special events. It is an attitude, a way of living that invites us to appreciate every moment, to find beauty in everyday life and to cultivate a sense of gratitude for the simple fact of existing. In a world that often seems obsessed with achievement and productivity, celebrating life reminds us that true value is not just in what we do or achieve, but in how we experience and enjoy each day. This chapter explores how we can adopt a mindset of daily celebration, what it really means to celebrate life, and how this perspective can transform our existence in a profound and lasting way.

For many people, the idea of celebrating life may seem abstract or reserved for special occasions. However, the celebration of life does not have to be limited to birthdays, weddings, or holidays. In fact, it can be a daily practice, a way to honor and value life as a whole, from the big moments to the smallest and seemingly insignificant ones. Celebrating life can be as simple as stopping to enjoy a hot cup of coffee in the morning, taking a moment to breathe deeply and feel the sun on your skin, or smiling at a stranger on the street.

These small acts of awareness and appreciation are, at their core, a celebration of life.

One of the keys to celebrating life is learning to be present. In the rush of everyday life, it is easy to get caught up in routine and overlook the moments of joy and beauty that are all around us. Being present means being fully in the here and now, without worrying about the past or the future. It is being aware of what is happening right now, both in your environment and within yourself. When you are present, you can notice and appreciate the small things that might otherwise go unnoticed: the singing of birds, the sound of rain, the laughter of a child. These moments, although simple, are opportunities to celebrate life as it is, in its purest and simplest form.

Gratitude is another essential component of celebrating life. Often, we are so focused on what we lack or what we want to achieve that we forget everything we already have. Practicing gratitude means taking time to recognize and be grateful for the big and small blessings that are a part of our lives. Whether you're grateful for your health, your family, your friends, or simply for waking up to a new day, gratitude connects you to the present and helps you see life from a perspective of abundance rather than shortage. This attitude of gratitude not only makes us happier, but also allows us to celebrate life in a deeper and more sincere way.

Another way to celebrate life is through the act of giving. Giving to others, whether it be time, attention, or resources, is a powerful way to connect with the broader meaning of life and experience joy that goes beyond personal satisfaction. When you give to others, you are not only improving their lives, but you are also strengthening your connection to the community and the world at large. This act of generosity is, in itself, a celebration of life, because it recognizes and honors the interconnectedness of all beings. By giving, we are celebrating the fact that we are part of something bigger than ourselves, something that deserves to be cared for and nurtured.

Celebrating life also involves accepting and embracing both moments of joy and challenges. Life is not perfect, and we all face hardships and losses at some point. However, even in these moments, it is possible to find reasons to celebrate. Celebrating life does not mean ignoring pain or sadness, but recognizing that these are also part of the human experience and that, in some way, they make us stronger and wiser. Accepting life's ups and downs with grace and gratitude is a way to celebrate resilience and the ability to grow and learn through adversity. This approach allows us to see life in its entirety, with all its contrasts, and appreciate beauty in its complexity.

Creativity also plays an important role in celebrating life. When we create, whether it be art, music, writing, or any other form of expression, we are celebrating life by shaping our thoughts, emotions, and experiences. Creativity allows us to connect with our deepest essence and share it with the world, which is, in itself, an act of celebration. Furthermore, the creative process invites us to explore and experiment, to leave our comfort zone and see the world with new eyes. Through creativity, we can discover new ways to celebrate life and find joy in the expression of who we are.

Another dimension of celebrating life is the cultivation of joy. Joy is not just an emotion, but a way of being, a choice we make every day. Cultivating joy means actively seeking out those things that make us happy and nourishing us, and making space for them in our lives. This can include activities we enjoy, such as spending time with loved ones, pursuing a hobby, or simply enjoying a walk outdoors. It can also mean surrounding ourselves with positive people who support us and inspire us to be the best version of ourselves. Joy is contagious, and when we cultivate it in our lives, we not only improve our own well-being, but we also radiate that positive energy to others.

Celebrating life also means honoring and caring for our bodies. Our body is the vehicle that allows us to experience all that life has to offer, and it deserves to be treated with respect and love. This means feeding him nutritious food, giving him the rest he needs, and keeping him active through movement that makes us feel good. Taking care of our body is a way to thank it for everything it does for us, and to celebrate life through health and well-being. Plus, when we feel good physically, it's easier to enjoy life and fully participate in all the activities and experiences we love.

Finally, celebrating life is a decision we make every day. It is a commitment to see the world with an attitude of wonder, gratitude and joy, and to look for the positive in every situation. It is a way of living that invites us to be aware of our blessings, to be present in every moment, and to enjoy the little things that make life beautiful. It is not about waiting for big events or changes to happen, but about finding reasons to celebrate in the everyday, in the simple, in what is often taken for granted.

In conclusion, celebrating life is an act of love and gratitude towards ourselves and the world around us. It is a daily practice that invites us to be present, to be grateful, to give, to be creative, and to cultivate joy. Through this mindset, we can transform our perception of life and find a deeper sense of satisfaction and happiness. Celebrating life not only makes us happier, but also helps us live more fully and meaningfully, recognizing and honoring the beauty that exists in each moment.